Larry,   10-20-14

Wishing you the best in life
& health —

        Dr. Thad Gala

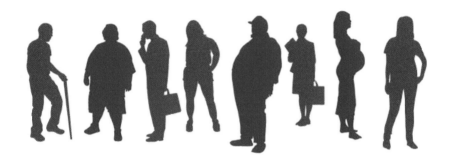

The *Secret*
to Defy
Disease and Decay

Thaddeus Gala, DC

Thaddeus Gala DC

The Secret to Defy Disease and Decay: Learn Why the American Diet is Killing You

Printed in the United States of America
First Printing 2014

ISBN 978-1-941780-00-8
www.DrThadGala.com

This book is for educational purposes only and not intended to replace the advice or recommendations of your physician. Talk to your physician before making any lifestyle changes.

The Secret To Defy Disease And Decay.

What is "The Secret to Defy Disease and Decay?" The concept for successfully understanding low-grade subclinical inflammation and how it drives pain, disease and weight gain is vital to success, yet often widely dismissed by current mainstream media, the layperson and medical professionals. As humans are typically reactive vs. proactive when it comes to their health, this behavior reinforces our current "health care system" that more closely represents a "sick care system." The vast majority of people do not go to the doctor until they have pain or a health concern. With this in mind, typical medical treatment is directed at reducing symptoms, not causes. While focusing and treating the symptoms may give a temporary false sense of security or improvement, the long-term result often leads to a progression, worsening and propagation of disease. This includes current and future health issues including weight gain, pain and arthritis, headaches, low energy, diabetes, heart disease, cancer, low energy, autoimmune issues and more.

Learning how to slow, stop and reverse aging.
There are many people that live long, quality, fulfilled and successful lives without giving a second thought to health in regards to physical, social or mental wellbeing. Conversely, others face seemingly insurmountable health issues that would challenge even the most steadfast of resolves with little traction or gain on health improvement. Ultimately, the quality and quantity of our life is dictated by when and how we make the decision to take action.

Facing the inevitable with grace.
While we can not live forever we can, however, at anytime dramatically improve our life experience by improving our Rising Health Potential. Typcially, the average person's health and quality of life diminshes with time and follows the blue line declining with age (see diagram to the right). The top gray line represents the aware and health conscious individual living and pursuing a highly productive, rewarding and quality life enriched with a sense of fullfillment. Thankfully, our bodies are extremely resiliant and can jump tracks at any time. While waiting to take action creates more Lost Health, I can attest from experience and supportive research, people in their 70's,

80's and 90's can still make substantial quality of life gains. Of course, those who start anti-inflammatory habits at a younger age experience higher and more pronounced positive outcomes by pursuing their Rising Health Potential and not waiting for chronic diease to set in.

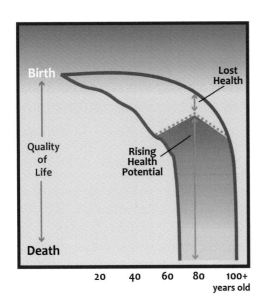

• We all have the potential to live a long, fulfilling, active and quality life until our final year or two with minimal physical limitations.

7

What is the difference and is there a clear answer to living a long and high quality life?
Why are some people healthy with minimal effort while others remain ill despite major investments of time and resources? Why do some feel "healthy" only to have a major health issue erupt seemingly out of nowhere? Myself, and many of the most advanced physicians, researchers and scientists now appreciate these health scenarios, including our current and future health, to be >90% dependent upon a single malleable and controllable factor: subclinical low grade inflammation.
This single factor is clearly understood to govern our health quality and happiness trajectory throughout our lifetime.

Quality of life and inflammation.
With low inflammation, people will typically experience a high quality of life with little to no medication reliance. As we make lifestyle choices that move us closer to high inflammation we notice a substantial reduction in quality of life, increased medication reliance and a corresponding risk of medication side effects (see diagram opposite page).

The big idea: Inflammation.
The sooner you understand this one idea for pursuing and maintaining health, the sooner you will increase your chances of a long fulfilling and quality life including:

- Increased Energy
- Improved Mental Clarity
- Enhanced Muscle Tone
- Weight Loss (or maintaining proper weight
- Normal Digestion & Bowel Function
- Reduction or Avoidance of Acute & Chronic Pain
- Faster Recovery From Travel/Workouts/Injury
- Abdominal Pain & G.E.R.D (Acid Reflux) Resolution.
- Reversal of O.S.A.S (Sleep Apnea & Snoring)
- Reduction of Chronic Disease: Heart, Cancer, Diabetes, Stroke, Arthritis, I.B.S., Fibromyalgia, Back Pain, RA/Lupus, Headaches, Acne, etc

Quality of life and inflammation.
With low inflammation, people will typically experience a high quality of life with little to no medication reliance. As we make lifestyle choices that move us closer to high inflammation we notice a substantial reduction in quality of life, increased medication reliance and a corresponding risk of medication side effects (see diagram opposite page).

10

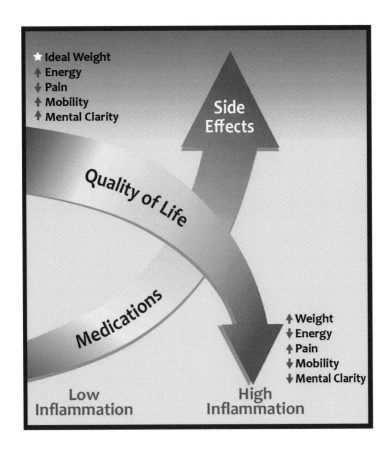

Inflammation: the lock and key

The single most powerful and easily influencing factor on our current and total health potential is increasingly and overwhelmingly recognized as subclinical inflammation. Inflammation is now understood to be the key driving force of chronic issues. Ailments or pain re-experienced or maintained >2wks are considered chronic, unnatural and typically mediated by low-grade subclinical inflammation.

What is inflammation?

Inflammation is the naturally occurring biochemical reaction that initiates the healing process following an insult to the body. Insults can include specific foods, stress, injury, toxins, etc. Typically, but not always, it involves pain or discomfort so our body knows something is damaged and needs both attention and protection. However, when short-term inflammation does not turn off and instead becomes chronic, this is unnatural. Chronic inflammation leads to

Note:
If you take 1 or more medications daily, including Aspirin, you have elevated inflammation. Additionally, if you have any chronic health frustrations you most likely suffer from inflammation.

problems that make life uncomfortable, bothersome and frustrating; while pain can be a symptom, it is not always present. Often, this absence of direct pain gives us a false sense of health security. We do not feel subclinical chronic inflammation progressing until we have an overt and negative health experience- such as a heart attack, cancer, stroke, diabetes, etc.

Clinical vs. subclinical inflammation.
We have all experienced clinical or acute inflammation. This obvious inflammation occurs after an injury, sunburn, mosquito or bug bite, etc. Typically this is short term and simply resolves quickly lasting <2wks. However, the opportunity for substantial health gains lies within understanding the concept of subclinical inflammation including its powerful and comprehensive influence. Keep in mind, we all have a certain amount of systemic subclinical inflammation, similar to lava below the earths surface, that rises and falls depending upon our daily life experiences and choices. Our inflammation levels can literally change minute to minute based on our current situation and choices. Some find this information frightening while many find it quite empowering. If the

pressure, or inflammation, in us builds overtime the likelihood of both major and minor overt disease eruption increases. The goal is to keep your subclinical inflammation as low as possible for as long as possible with healthy lifestyle choices. We will discuss the influencers of inflammation when we review the keystones for reversing and lowering subclinical inflammation.

hs-CRP: The power to predict your future.
While there are many tests for subclinical inflammation, since about 2002 to present, an hs-CRP blood test has been considered the single most influential marker in measuring and monitoring disease risk and progression. hs-CRP should not be confused with ESR or CRP and can be performed by your health care provider. hs-CRP is produced in the liver in response to noxious stimulus to the body including being overweight, infection, specific inflammatory foods, sedentary activities, and smoking, to name a few. The goal is to have this marker as low as possible for as long as possible without the use of artificial chemical or external agents such as statins, NSAIDS or other anti-inflammatory drugs. Daily anti-inflammatory choices will have the most lasting and powerful positive

impact on hs-CRP. Similar to the rise and fall of lava below the earth's surface, measuring hs-CRP is a predictive tool for disease. When inflammation gets high, we experience disease or discomfort.

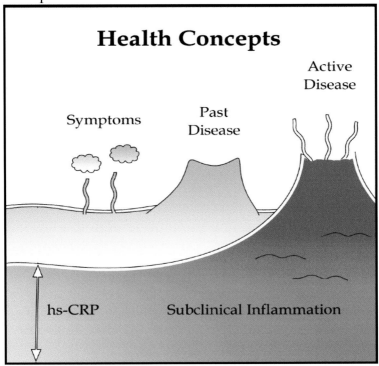

Symptom vs. cause.

Pursuing health and an anti-inflammatory lifestyle requires the ability to understand the difference between symptoms and cause. While this understanding is easy in theory, daily life experiences are not always clear-cut. For instance, when you step on a dog's tail (root cause) and it barks (symptom), you would not put a muzzle on the dog to stop the barking (symptom). Clearly, the best resolution is removing the foot from the dogs tail (root cause). Similarly, cutting a weed (symptom) at the base vs digging up the root is consistent with mainstream and traditional medicine treating symptoms with medications and surgeries rather than root causes. Unfortunately, if the root cause is never fully addressed by treating superficial symptoms, we typically promote an ongoing illusion of the need for daily medication reliance. That is, medications dealing with blood pressure, cholesterol, diabetes, chronic pain, etc, do not effectively treat the root cause, which is why daily usage must continue until the true problem is addressed. This true cause is now increasingly recognized as subclinical inflammation and spans all chronic diseases including Obstructive Sleep Apnea Syndrome (OSAS), migraines, TMJ, joint stiffness, cramps, Polycystic Ovarian

Syndrome (PCOS), cancer, heart disease, diabetes and auto-immune issues to name a few.

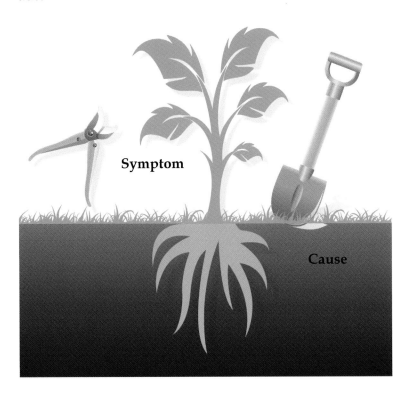

Symptom

Cause

Superficial vs. basal causes with "Perpetual Why."
After understanding the concept of focusing on Causes vs. Symptoms, you can look even deeper to focus on the most powerful of levers for lasting and comprehensive health improvement of lowering inflammation. The idea is to continue asking "Why" until you believe you uncover the true root cause of the inflammation.

The "Perpetual Why" in motion.
The following Q&A method can be used to find causative agents not only with undesirable health symptoms but in business, relationship or other areas of your life. This tool is considered the "Perpetual Why" and within each answer is the subsequent question followed by the next why. The following example could be used for any chronic issue related to health including pain, headaches, TMJ, heart disease, poor skin quality, etc. For best results, be sure each answer is phrased as an "I" statement to empower yourself to make a change. If you do not phrase or reword the answer as an "I" statement, you may become paralyzed in taking meaningful action and become mentally powerless. This technique will help you from succumbing to the idea that external forces are controlling

your health and instead put you in a position of correcting the root cause.

Question or Why	Answer
Why do I have chronic pain?	I have inflammation.
Why do I have inflammation?	I eat inflammatory foods.
Why do I eat inflammatory foods?	I want to eat something quickly
Why do I eat something quickly?	I have a busy work week.
Why don't I plan ahead?	I like to watch TV on Sunday.

Q. Why don't I set aside time on Sunday to plan for a healthy week?
A. (True Why Discovered) Make it a priority to set aside time.

Of course, you can stop at any level of the "Perpetual Why" if it is believed taking action at that level will fix the root cause.

Understanding your health frustrations.
While most people are able to articulate their financial, business or other tangible goals, many are not able to clearly articulate personal goals including the setting of defined and measurable health outcomes. Simply put, to find your health goals identify first what frustrates you. When viewed in reverse this exercise provides the emotional framework for identifying your logical next steps in goal achievement.

Frustrations = Goals
As a quick exercise take 2-5 min right now to write down your frustrations. Then, reverse the concept to outline your goals. This is a great tool. You will quickly find this approach can be used in any aspect of life to promote improvement and satisfaction. Be sure to use the "Perpetual Whys" to identify and outline the true baseline and next step to lead you towards the biggest impact in goal achievement.

Frustration/Emotion	Goal/Logic
→I Don't Like Being Fat	→Lose 25+lbs
→I Am Tired Of Low Energy	→Lower Inflammation
→I Dislike Taking Drugs	→Find Drugless Physicians
→I Don't Like Chronic Pain	→Lower Inflammation
→My Skin Is Saggy	→Exercise 15min daily

Of course, nearly every goal should include the action step of lowering inflammation. Once your goals are established, quickly move to implementing meaningful action steps.

The 0 medication myth.
Some people believe that because they either do not take or have disbanded medications, their body is healthy. While medications do have side effects, elimination without focusing on inflammation can potentially be even more harmful from rebound effects. If you are on medications, as with blood sugar medications for diabetes, once you start to lower your inflammation and blood sugar levels you can typically start to safely stair step off your medications in several weeks with the help of your prescribing physician. It has been our experience with clients and patients that the overwhelming majority of chronic issues normalize with elimination of chronic medications in 1-8 months of following an anti-inflammatory lifestyle.

This conceptual scenario shows how we work with clients in reversing diabetes and can conceptually be used for cholesterol, blood pressure, pain and other chronic medications with the aid of a physician.

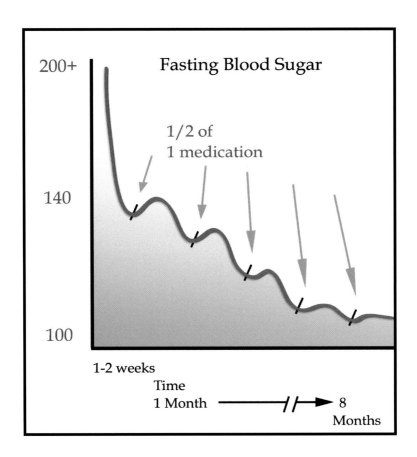

We all decide: either sooner or later.
Many outwardly appearing healthy people claim, "I have done XYZ habit my entire life and look at how healthy I am!" Conversely, many sick people lament, "If I had only taken better care of myself when I was younger." Sadly, these two statements often go hand in hand. Thankfully, it is never too late to take action. I can attest from years of experience working with parents and babies all the way through to those in their nineties, that most, if not all people, are capable of making substantial health gains with several simple yet keystone lifestyle changes. People successful in life, business and health typically take quick and decisive action in formulating new habits so they can layer the added benefits of the next healthy habit. Focus on your goals and you will soon be enjoying the freedom to enjoy a happier, healthier and higher quality life.

Health is not merely the absence of disease.
Now that you are obtaining this information, you will find many people need help in understanding the destructive power of subclinical inflammation. Feeling fine does not equate to being healthy. We now appreciate the power of the long term, sometimes subtle, underlying causation of weight gain, health frustrations and disease being linked to the smoldering irritant of chronic low-grade inflammation we all have to varying degrees.

Health is not merely being thin.
Most people want and need to lose weight. While reducing inflammation has been demonstrated to be one of the best long-term weight loss methods, what about people who are thin or normal weight? Many people erroneously associate being a healthy weight with being healthy. This dangerous assumption often causes people to miss the connection between inflammation and disease progression. Again, without addressing low-grade inflammation, outwardly appearing thin or healthy individuals can easily suffer from chronic conditions including, fatigue, irregular bowel function, asthma, allergies, headaches, chronic pain, fibromyalgia and autoimmune conditions to name a few.

The 13 Keystones To Lower Inflammation

The Ultimate Goal.
The ultimate goal is to quickly and effectively establish a
framework of daily habits that reinforce an anti-
inflammatory lifestyle.

Keystone #1
Improve your odds by lowering inflammation.
One of the first steps is getting a clear baseline of your inflammation. While testing for inflammation is a growing field, the single and biggest predictive test is currently recognized as hs-CRP. While a staggering 50% of heart attacks occur in people with normal cholesterol, myself and other researchers now recognize that nearly all cases of chronic disease, cancer and heart attacks are consistently accompanied by preexisting elevated subclinical inflammation.

hs-CRP Blood Test Risk Ranges:

Low risk: less than	1.0mg/L
Medium risk:	1-3.0mg/L
High risk: above	3.0-10mg/L
Extreme or Acute risk: over	10mg/L

Many researchers are now finding a healthy hs-CRP is below 0.5 and even below 0.1 as being ideal. For years, my hs-CRP has been consistently under 0.1 once I understood the inflammatory concept and began self testing while concurrently integrating the following keystone habits.

We now know elevated low grade inflammation promotes everything from Multiple Sclerosis, heart disease and cancer to diabetes, chronic pain, arthritis, constipation/diarrhea and low energy.

Note:
Do not let all your decisions rest on hs-CRP. While a positive test is the best for measuring subclinical inflammation, a low or negative test does not guarantee low inflammation. It can only confirm high inflammation and lend guidance in understanding how your lifestyle decisions are impacting your body's chemistry in accelerating or slowing aging and disease manifestation. Other inflammatory tests exist. However, these tests are typically less sensitive in predictive value when compared with hs-CRP.

Ideal vs actual.
Ideally, you want your blood test of hs-CRP undetectable and under 0.1. While 1.0 is typically difficult to obtain, in actuality, most people can get their hs-CRP quite low and below 1.0.

Keystone #2
Improve your understanding of the 20:1 ratios.

Most researchers agree that a substantial portion of our inflammation is governed by Essential Fatty Acid (EFAs – omega-3, 6 & 9) consumption. Our bodies are incapable of producing these fats intrinsically and therefore, we are completely dependent upon dietary sources for these essential nutrients. It is important to recognize the difference and power of these fats. While most people have heard of the omega-3 fats found in fish, wild game and green leafy vegetables, many people do not understand the power of omega-6 in its promotion of chronic disease. In short, omega-3 fats turn inflammation off while omega-6 fats turn inflammation on. In lay terms, this translates to foods containing omega-6 fats as perpetrators of disease and pain. Most people with low inflammation have a ratio range of omega-6:omega-3 around 1:1 to 4:1. However, the average person is usually inflamed to the degree of 10:1 to as high as 20:1 in many cases. This means the typical person is 10-20X's more inflamed than they should be by health standards. Omega-6 fats are especially to be avoided if you want to reverse or prevent chronic disease including diabetes, chronic pain, fibromyalgia, osteoporosis or have a desire to improve brain function and cognition. Lastly, omega-9 fats are typically anti-inflammatory and found in olive oil, many nuts and avocados.

Foods to avoid: Inflammatory omega-6
The following foods are important to reduce or eliminate altogether in the diet:

- Grains & Wheat Products
- Cereals, Pastas, Breads & Bagels
- Beans, Legumes & Lentils
- Seeds & Seed Oils
- Corn & Corn Oil
- Sesame, Sunflower, Soy & Peanut Oil
- Grain Finished Fatty Meat
- Farm Raised Fish
- Most Processed Oils
- Packaged Foods

Keystone #3
Improve your consumption of omega-3 fats.
As discussed, equally important as reducing the pro-inflammatory omega-6 fats is increasing anti-inflammatory omega-3 fats. Omega-3 fats have been linked to improved skin quality, reduced pain, heart health and reduction of auto-immune conditions to name a few.

Foods to include: Anti-inflammatory omega-3
The following foods are important to increase in the diet:
- Wild Fish
- Wild Game
- Green Leafy Vegetables
- Grass Finished Meats
- Walnuts
- Omega-3 Eggs
- Omega-3 Supplementation (Fish or Krill Oil)

Keystone #4
Improve your ability to appreciate a grain imbalance.
While most people have heard of gluten as related to wheat and grains including the associated health consequences, few have heard of the other inflammatory components still present in gluten free products. These inflammatory chemicals are equally powerful in causing headaches, arthritis, diabetes, chronic pain, low energy, cognitive decline, mental fog, I.B.S., bloating diarrhea and chronic disease. It is important to recognize that grains and most seeds increase tissue acidity, are indigestible in the raw form, are high in omega-6 fats, contain phytic acid, promote weight gain, strain the pancreas (promoting diabetes), activate zonulin, are a poor source of fiber, contain WGA and are a poor source of micronutrients. These aforementioned inflammatory chemicals are designed to protect the seed by detouring predators (humans) with sickness to detour future preference. Many people do not draw this direct conclusion as the cause and effect can be delayed from hours to years.

Foods to avoid:
- Grains, Wheat & Seeds
- Beans, Corn & Legumes
- Quinoa & Lentils
- Oats, Barley, Rice, Etc.

Keystone #5
Improve your understanding of dairy.
Nearly everyday more research sheds light on the harmful health consequences of dairy consumption in any form. We now appreciate the top offenders of dairy to include harmful insulin effects, being a poor source of calcium and vitamin D and containing the problematic sugar lactose, to name a few. Cow's milk has been linked to type I diabetes, multiple sclerosis, ulcerative colitis and Crohn's disease. Further, dairy contains many hormones that are unnatural for human exposure including, betacellulin (BTC), insulin like growth factor 1 (IGF-1) and estrogens. Nearly 70+ hormones have been identified in dairy products with many containing the inherent ability to cross the intestinal membrane resulting in potentially harmful health outcomes upon entering the blood stream. Dairy is considered one of the leading causative agents in autoimmune disorders and the chronic inflammatory process. Reducing or avoiding all forms of dairy is considered best practice for reducing inflammation.

Keystone #6
Improve your ability to deal with conflict.
Conflict and stress are a way of life and necessary for survival. Stress prompts us to remedy or leave an unhealthy environment. We now know that inflammation is not only governed by dietary sources but by our mental state and stress levels. When we are stressed, overworked, argumentative or taxed without a reasonably quick resolution, we create a chronic elevation of our subclinical inflammation. The power of the mind in reducing or elevating inflammation is increasingly understood as paramount in the disease process. Look for common and uncommon sources of stress in your life and work diligently to remove as many as possible in conjunction with implementing healthy stress resolution practices. In addition to accelerating the disease and inflammatory process, specifically, stress can result in acne, psoriasis, warts, heart disease, I.B.S, cancer, headaches and cognitive decline to name a few.

Lower conflict inflammation:
- Exercise, Walk, Massage
- Nature Experiences & Vistas
- Breaks From Arguments
- Laughing & Meditation
- Reading a Favorite Book
- Undistracted Quality Time with Friends & Family

Keystone #7
Improve your chances of a win.
Waiting until the last minute often offers little opportunity for healthy anti-inflammatory decisions. Catering to our often busy lives, society has unintentionally fostered enhanced accessibility to an inflammatory lifestyle. The ease of quickly satisfying hunger in today's busy lifestyle is why pro-inflammatory boxed and canned foods are prevalent. A bit of foresight and planning can go a long way in creating healthy habits in avoiding this inflammatory trap. People destined for disease often find excuses as to why they cannot make healthy food and lifestyle choices a priority while healthy people navigate the same world empowered. Successful people plan and prepare ahead making an anti-inflammatory lifestyle a way of life and daily practice. The quicker you adopt this empowerment mindset, the sooner you can start to reverse the inflammatory disease progression including the aging process.

Invest in your schedule:
- Set a daily, weekly and monthly schedule that caters to integrating healthy habits.

Keystone #8
Improve your key nutrients.

Many people are overfed and undernourished. Meaning, we take in too many calories without enough nutrients. The key is to eat nutrient dense foods low on the glycemic index. Colorful vegetables and fruits contain many natural anti-oxidants. Shoot for a variety every day. If weight or blood sugar is an issue, reduce fruit consumption and increase vegetable and lean protein intake. Most people have heard of vitamins and minerals. However, research shows an increasingly recognized number of compounds and anti-inflammatory benefits from specific plants including the location grown, color, soil, light conditions and culinary preparation. The key is to focus on as many colorful varieties of vegetables with occasional fruit as possible. Anti-inflammatory chemicals found in plants help reduce inflammation and offer protection from sunburn and free radical damage, aging, chronic pain, arthritis, disc herniation and aid in lowering cholesterol.

Foods to include:
- Vegetables & Berries of all colors
- Minimally Cooked Meats
- Herbs and Spices

Keystone #9
Improve your ability to shed fat and lower inflammation with supplements.

Key nutrients with supplementation added to a healthy anti-inflammatory diet are paramount in reducing the inflammatory process and turning your body into an efficient and effective fat burning furnace. Successful people view supplements as an adjunct, not a replacement for an anti-inflammatory lifestyle. Proper supplement dosage is vital for effectiveness. While specific conditions should be addressed with a health care professional, there are many other effective supplements not listed below that are condition specific including chromium with antioxidants for diabetes and turmeric for Alzheimer's. Below are ranges and again, should be discussed with a health care professional before making any changes.

- Omega-3: 2-3,000mg combined EPA/DHA
- Iron Free Multi-Vitamin
- Vitamin D: 5,000-25,000IU daily
- Magnesium: 300-1000mg daily
- Calcium 300-1,000mg daily
- Probiotics

Keystone #10
Improve your ability to eliminate sugar.
Sugar is linked to nearly every disease. Most oncologists will confirm: Sugar = Cancer. Sugar not only contributes to adiposity (fat) but also accelerates the aging and disease process. Sugar consumption stimulates insulin, which has been shown to promote diabetes, PCOS, skin tags, obesity, headaches, acne as well as activating and reinforcing addictive neurological pathways in the brain.

Foods to avoid:
- Potatoes, Starch, Grains
- Dried Fruit
- Juice & Soda
- Candy
- Limit Fresh Fruit to 3 or Less Servings Daily

Note:
If you are overweight or diabetic, less than 1 or 2 servings of fruit a day may be necessary until reaching your health goals.

Keystone #11
Improve your daily exercise.

Start with small wins. If you sit all day and it is difficult to walk, start by getting in and out of your chair 10x's by going from sitting to standing every 4 hours. If you are able to walk, try walking at least 10 minutes every day working up to 10 minutes of vigorous walking 3-5 times a week if you can. If you are able to jog, try to jog for 15 minutes 3-5 times a week with intermittent fast 15 second runs every 5 minutes or so. Exercise will help fast track disease reversal and healing. Exercise forces inflammatory disease causing chemicals out of your body more quickly than sitting. Of the three components to exercise: intensity, frequency and duration, intensity is the most important. This means it is better to do more intense short workouts totaling 15 minutes vs. 60 plus minutes at low intensity.

Exercise 5-15min total:
High Intensity with Short Duration is better than Low Intensity with Long Duration.
The idea is to get the heart rate up for short bursts.

Keystone #12
Improve your water consumption.
Low grade dehydration affects mental and physical performance dramatically. A general rule is to drink up to half your body weight in ounces (oz) a day. So if you weigh 200lbs, you need to drink up to 100oz of water which is the equivalent 1.5 gallons daily. I encourage people to fill up a jug or bottles with the total they need to drink each day and place on either their kitchen counter or work station. This allows for a visual indicator of keeping you on track. Water is important for helping your cells and body flush out inflammatory chemicals and replace it with the anti-inflammatory chemicals you are now incorporating.

Water intake basic formula:
Body Weight ÷ 2 = Total oz Daily

Gallons per day
Total oz ÷ by 64 = Total Daily Gallons

Glasses per day
Total oz ÷ 8 = Total 8oz Daily Glasses

Keystone #13
Improve your internal and external waistline.
Most people are aware of the health risks associated with being overweight. We now know adipose (fat) is actually considered its own endocrine organ and will pump inflammation directly into the blood stream. Worse yet, we now know your Internal Waistline (visceral or fat around your internal organs) can be equally detrimental. Not only is being overweight detrimental to self-image and mental stress, the inflammation it injects into the blood promotes the disease cycle. Thankfully, following the other Keystones in this book will help you thin your Internal and External Waistlines quickly. It is not uncommon to lose 5-30+lbs in a single month following these Keystones.

Strategies for long term success.
Means. Motivation. Knowledge

Most people have the means to purchase food and live an anti-inflammatory lifestyle. Your Motivation comes from your desire to overcome your health frustrations and reach your goals. Knowledge of inflammatory mediators is ongoing. Motivation and knowledge are where many people fall short. If this is you, do not be discouraged. Just knowing the key factors that cause inflammation does not translate to seamless lifestyle integration. Empower yourself by taking a critical look at each of these three areas and take the necessary action steps to improve until you reach your goals. If you find yourself short on any of the three areas, a coaching support program can provide the tools to identify key action steps. As mentioned earlier, answering: "What frustrates me about my current health?" is a good starting point to identify your goals. These goals should be looked at regularly for encouragement. If you need help on how to integrate healthy eating habits, research or find a coach and support system with successful experience.

Steps to success:
- Means
- Motivation
- Knowledge

43

"If you fail to plan, you plan to fail"
Benjamin Franklin

There are many sources of inflammation that are necessary to address for appropriate weight loss, disease prevention and reversal. Nutrition is one of the most common. Dr. Gala and the team at The Institute for Natural Disease Reversal help people identify the true cause of inflammation. In addition, they help to formulate clear and easy action steps for individualized and self-sustaining habits to mitigate, prevent and reverse health issues. The most successful people benefit from working with an experienced coach in outlining and implementing a clear and individualized day-to-day autopilot system of easy action steps. This helps people make a reality of reversing health frustrations and achieving their health goals in 1-8 months.

Lastly, many medications can cause focused nutritional deficiencies. In addition to coaching and daily support, The Institute For Natural Disease Reversal provides detailed descriptions of what supplements individuals may benefit from to mitigate medication side effects and promote nutritional balance in the body to help lower inflammation.

The Institute For Natural Disease Reversal
The goal of Dr. Thaddeus Gala and The Institute for Natural Disease Reversal is to help people prevent and reverse inflammation and chronic health issues in 1-8 months so they can avoid, reduce or completely eliminate medication reliance. By integrating short and long term habits for self management, individuals can pursue a long and high quality life.

If you are interested in learning more about support, resources, or personal health coaching, please contact us at:

www.DrThadGala.com
Support@DrThadGala.com

To assess your personal inflammation score in additional areas of health, including an online quiz and custom report, learn more with a self-assessment at:

DrThadGala.com